Gluten-Free Grocery List and Food

Embracing Variety: Incorporating Ethnic Flavors and Global Cuisine into Gluten-Free Eating

McDonnell B. Young

Table of Contents

Introduction

Emma had always been an enthusiastic cook. Her kitchen was her sanctuary, a place where she crafted meals with love and creativity. But when she was diagnosed with celiac disease, her culinary world was suddenly filled with challenges. The joy of cooking became overshadowed by the stress of navigating a gluten-free diet.

For months, Emma struggled to make sense of which foods were safe and which were not. She found herself staring at grocery store shelves, overwhelmed by confusing labels and hidden sources of gluten. The fun of meal planning had turned into a daily battle against invisible gluten lurking in processed foods.

One day, while browsing online for a solution, Emma stumbled upon a guide titled "Gluten-Free Grocery List and Food." Intrigued, she clicked to learn more. What she discovered was a comprehensive tool designed precisely for people like her, who needed clarity and confidence in their gluten-free journey.

The guide promised to take the guesswork out of shopping. It offered a detailed list of gluten-free foods to eat, categorized by fresh fruits and vegetables, proteins, dairy alternatives, grains, and more. Emma was impressed by how meticulously it separated safe options from those to avoid, including the often-overlooked hidden sources of gluten. This was exactly what she needed—clear, actionable information that would save her countless hours of research.

The guide didn't stop there. It included practical advice on reading labels, understanding gluten-free certifications, and avoiding cross-contamination. Emma found the sections on meal planning and budgeting particularly valuable. The sample meal plans were not only practical but also inspiring, showing her how to create delicious and varied meals without feeling restricted.

With her newfound knowledge, Emma felt a wave of relief. The guide had transformed her approach to grocery shopping and meal planning. She no longer felt lost in the aisles of her local store. Instead, she walked confidently, her shopping cart filled with safe and satisfying foods.

Emma's kitchen once again became a place of joy. With the help of the guide, she was able to explore new recipes, enjoy the foods she loved, and even share her culinary creations with friends and family. Her gluten-free journey, once fraught with uncertainty, had become an adventure filled with delicious possibilities.

Emma's story is a testament to the value of the "Gluten-Free Grocery List and Food" guide. It's more than just a list; it's a companion for anyone navigating the complexities of a gluten-free lifestyle. For anyone feeling overwhelmed by gluten-free grocery shopping, this guide offers the clarity and support needed to turn challenges into opportunities for culinary creativity and enjoyment.

Understanding Gluten and Its Impact

Gluten is a complex protein found in wheat, barley, and rye, which plays a crucial role in giving dough its elasticity and helping it rise. When gluten is present in foods, it contributes to the texture and chewiness that many baked goods possess. For individuals with celiac disease, gluten is a harmful substance that triggers an autoimmune response. This response damages the small intestine's lining, leading to a range of symptoms such as abdominal pain, diarrhea, and fatigue. Consequently, for those with celiac disease, a strict gluten-free diet is essential to manage symptoms and prevent long-term health issues.

Gluten sensitivity or non-celiac gluten sensitivity (NCGS) is another condition where individuals experience discomfort after consuming gluten, although they do not have celiac disease or wheat allergy. Symptoms of NCGS can include bloating, stomach pain, and headaches, which can significantly impact one's quality of life. Unlike celiac disease, NCGS does not cause damage to the intestine but still necessitates a gluten-free diet to alleviate symptoms. For those affected by NCGS, understanding which foods contain gluten is critical for managing their health and well-being.

Understanding the impact of gluten on health is vital for anyone embarking on a gluten-free diet. Gluten can be found in a wide array of processed foods beyond obvious sources like bread and pasta. It is often used as a stabilizing or thickening agent in sauces, soups, and even some medications. This makes navigating a gluten-free lifestyle particularly challenging, as hidden gluten can be present in seemingly innocuous products. The complexity of identifying gluten in various food items underscores the importance of having a comprehensive guide to make informed choices.

A gluten-free grocery list is an indispensable tool for anyone adhering to a gluten-free diet. It simplifies the process of selecting safe foods by providing a clear and organized list of items that are free from gluten. This list typically includes fresh produce, unprocessed proteins, and gluten-free grains, all of which can be enjoyed without concern. It also highlights foods to avoid, such as those containing wheat, barley, or rye, along with processed foods where gluten might be an ingredient. Having such a guide can significantly reduce the stress and confusion associated with gluten-free shopping.

For individuals newly diagnosed with celiac disease or those with gluten sensitivities, the transition to a gluten-free diet can be overwhelming. The sheer volume of information and the need to read labels meticulously can be daunting. A well-structured gluten-free grocery list helps mitigate this challenge by consolidating essential information into one accessible format. This guide serves not only as a shopping tool but also as an educational resource, helping individuals understand which foods are safe and how to avoid potential sources of gluten.

The impact of gluten on individuals with celiac disease or gluten sensitivity emphasizes the need for careful dietary management. Eating foods that contain gluten, even in small amounts, can lead to adverse health effects and prolonged discomfort. Therefore, a gluten-free grocery list and food guide become crucial resources for maintaining health and preventing symptoms. By offering clarity on what foods to include and what to avoid, this guide empowers individuals to make informed choices, ensuring that their dietary needs are met effectively.

Ultimately, the journey towards a gluten-free lifestyle is greatly facilitated by having access to a detailed and reliable guide. Understanding the role of gluten and its impact on health underscores the importance of using such resources to navigate dietary restrictions with confidence. Whether for managing a medical condition or improving overall well-being, a gluten-free grocery list serves as a valuable ally, making the pursuit of a healthy, gluten-free life more manageable and less stressful.

The Importance of a Gluten-Free Diet

A gluten-free diet is crucial for individuals with celiac disease, a condition in which consuming gluten—a protein found in wheat, barley, and rye—triggers an immune response that damages the small intestine. This damage impairs nutrient absorption and can lead to a variety of severe health issues, including malnutrition, anemia, and bone density loss. For those with celiac disease, avoiding gluten is not a choice but a necessity to maintain their health and well-being.

The significance of a gluten-free diet extends beyond just celiac disease. Many people experience non-celiac gluten sensitivity, where gluten intake can cause discomfort and symptoms such as bloating, fatigue, and headaches. While not as severe as celiac disease, managing gluten sensitivity through a strict gluten-free diet can greatly improve the quality of life for these individuals. A well-planned gluten-free diet helps to alleviate these symptoms and supports overall health.

Navigating the gluten-free landscape can be challenging without proper guidance, especially when it comes to grocery shopping. Gluten is present in many processed and packaged foods, often hidden under various names and forms. This complexity makes it essential for individuals on a gluten-free diet to be vigilant about what they purchase and consume. A comprehensive gluten-free grocery list helps streamline this process by clearly identifying safe foods and avoiding potential sources of gluten.

A thoughtfully designed gluten-free grocery list provides clarity and convenience by categorizing foods into those that are safe and those to avoid. It includes fresh fruits and vegetables, gluten-free grains, dairy and dairy alternatives, and proteins, ensuring that individuals can maintain a balanced and nutritious diet without inadvertently consuming gluten. This organization not only simplifies shopping but also helps in planning meals that adhere to gluten-free guidelines.

Moreover, a well-curated list aids in preventing cross-contamination, a common issue that can occur when gluten-free foods come into contact with gluten-containing items. Understanding how to avoid cross-contamination is essential for individuals with celiac disease or severe gluten sensitivity. The grocery list serves as a tool for identifying not just inherently gluten-free foods, but also those that have been processed or handled in ways that minimize contamination risks.

The benefits of following a gluten-free diet are evident in improved digestive health, enhanced energy levels, and overall better quality of life. For those managing gluten-related disorders, adhering to a gluten-free diet can lead to a dramatic reduction in symptoms and a more stable health condition. By leveraging a well-prepared gluten-free grocery list, individuals can ensure they are consistently making choices that align with their dietary needs.

In essence, a gluten-free grocery list is more than just a convenience; it is a critical resource for anyone who needs to adhere to a gluten-free diet. It helps demystify the shopping process, supports proper meal planning, and ultimately contributes to maintaining a healthy and balanced diet. For those navigating the complexities of gluten-free living, this guide is an invaluable asset in achieving a healthier, symptom-free lifestyle.

How to Use This Guide

When embarking on a gluten-free journey, the "Gluten-Free Grocery List and Food" guide becomes an essential tool in ensuring a safe and enjoyable dietary experience. To effectively use this guide, start by familiarizing yourself with the key sections that outline which foods are safe and which should be avoided. This knowledge will empower you to make informed choices as you navigate through grocery store aisles, avoiding the confusion and uncertainty that often accompany a gluten-free diet.

Begin by examining the detailed lists of gluten-free foods provided. These sections categorize various types of foods, such as fruits, vegetables, proteins, and grains, into clear, easy-to-follow categories. Understanding these categories will help you build a well-rounded shopping list that aligns with your dietary needs. As you become more accustomed to these lists, you'll gain confidence in selecting products that adhere to your gluten-free requirements.

Next, pay close attention to the guidance on reading food labels. The guide offers practical advice on identifying gluten-free products, including tips on spotting hidden sources of gluten that may not be immediately obvious. This is crucial for avoiding common pitfalls and ensuring that you only consume safe products. Learning how to read labels effectively will streamline your shopping process and reduce the risk of accidental gluten exposure.

The guide also provides valuable insights into cross-contamination, a critical aspect of maintaining a strict gluten-free diet. Understanding how cross-contamination can occur and the steps to prevent it will help you create a safe cooking environment. This includes being mindful of shared kitchen utensils and surfaces, which is essential for keeping gluten from contaminating your meals.

In addition to practical advice on food selection and preparation, the guide includes sample meal plans and budgeting tips. These resources are designed to simplify meal planning and make it more enjoyable. By following the suggested meal plans, you can explore a variety of gluten-free recipes and ensure that your diet remains balanced and nutritious. The budgeting tips will help you manage costs while still enjoying a diverse range of gluten-free foods.

Utilize the guide's list of recommended gluten-free brands and products to further enhance your shopping experience. These recommendations are based on thorough research and can serve as a starting point for discovering reliable gluten-free options. By incorporating these brands into your shopping routine, you can save time and reduce the risk of purchasing products that may not meet your dietary needs.

Finally, embrace the guide as an ongoing resource rather than a one-time reference. As you gain experience with your gluten-free diet, revisit the guide to refresh your knowledge and explore new sections. The more you engage with the guide, the more proficient you will become in managing your gluten-free lifestyle, ultimately transforming it from a challenge into a rewarding and enjoyable experience.

Chapter 1: Essentials of a Gluten-Free Diet

What is Gluten?

Gluten is a group of proteins found in wheat, barley, and rye, which are commonly used in many foods. It plays a crucial role in giving dough its elasticity and helping it rise, which is why gluten-containing grains are often used in baking. When flour is mixed with water, gluten proteins form a network that traps air bubbles, resulting in the chewy texture of bread and other baked goods. This property makes gluten integral to many traditional recipes and processed foods.

For individuals with celiac disease or gluten sensitivity, consuming gluten can trigger adverse reactions. Celiac disease is an autoimmune disorder where the ingestion of gluten leads to inflammation and damage in the small intestine. This damage impairs nutrient absorption and can result in a variety of gastrointestinal and systemic symptoms. Gluten sensitivity, on the other hand, may not cause intestinal damage but can lead to symptoms like bloating, headaches, and fatigue upon consuming gluten-containing foods.

Understanding what gluten is and where it is found is crucial for anyone needing to avoid it. Gluten is present in obvious sources such as bread, pasta, and baked goods, but it can also be hidden in less obvious products like sauces, soups, and processed foods. Gluten acts as a stabilizer or thickening agent in many processed foods, so it's essential to scrutinize ingredient lists and labels carefully to avoid accidental exposure.

The guide provides detailed information on how to identify gluten in various foods, highlighting the importance of being vigilant about ingredient lists. It also explains how gluten can be present in modified food starches, malt, and other additives that may not explicitly mention gluten but still pose a risk. This level of detail helps readers make informed decisions while shopping, ensuring that they select products that are truly gluten-free.

It's also important to understand that cross-contamination can occur when gluten-free foods come into contact with gluten-containing products or surfaces. This can happen in shared kitchens or when using common utensils. The guide emphasizes the need for careful food preparation practices to prevent cross-contamination, which is crucial for maintaining a strict gluten-free diet and avoiding unintended gluten exposure.

Gluten-free diets often require substituting traditional grains with alternatives like rice, quinoa, and gluten-free oats. These substitutes not only avoid gluten but also offer nutritional benefits. The guide helps readers navigate these alternatives by providing a comprehensive list of safe grains and flours, ensuring that individuals following a gluten-free diet can still enjoy a variety of foods without sacrificing nutrition or taste.

Overall, understanding what gluten is and its role in food production is fundamental to managing a gluten-free diet effectively. The guide aims to educate readers on these aspects, providing practical advice and resources to help them identify and avoid gluten in their daily food choices. This knowledge is essential for maintaining health and well-being while adhering to a gluten-free lifestyle.

Common Sources of Gluten

Gluten, a protein found in certain grains, is a key concern for anyone following a gluten-free diet. Understanding its common sources is crucial for managing dietary needs and preventing accidental gluten ingestion. Wheat is the most prominent source of gluten and is found in a variety of products, from bread and pasta to baked goods and cereals. Beyond the obvious bread and pasta, wheat is also used in less apparent forms such as wheat flour, wheat bran, and wheat germ, which can be included in many processed foods.

Another major gluten-containing grain is barley, which is often used in malt products. Barley is commonly found in malted beverages like beer, as well as in malt flavorings and malt extracts used in many processed foods. Its presence in these products can make it challenging to avoid unless you are vigilant in checking ingredient lists and labels. Barley is also used in some cereals and soups, so attention to detail is necessary when evaluating food options.

Rye, another grain that contains gluten, is typically used in rye bread, rye crackers, and some cereals. Its use can sometimes be less obvious as it may be included in mixed-grain products or used as a flavoring agent. As with wheat and barley, careful label reading is essential to identify rye in various foods and ensure it's avoided in a gluten-free diet.

Oats, while naturally gluten-free, are often contaminated with gluten during processing because they are frequently processed in facilities that handle wheat, barley, or rye. Some brands offer certified gluten-free oats, which are processed in dedicated facilities, making them safe for those with celiac disease or severe gluten sensitivity. Choosing oats labeled as gluten-free is essential to avoid contamination and adhere to a strict gluten-free diet.

Gluten can also be present in various food additives and processed ingredients. For instance, modified food starch, often used as a thickening agent, can be derived from gluten-containing grains. Maltodextrin, another common additive, is usually gluten-free but should be scrutinized if derived from wheat. It's important to be cautious with processed foods, as gluten can be hidden in ingredients that are not immediately recognizable as gluten-containing.

Cross-contamination is another critical issue when managing a gluten-free diet. Even trace amounts of gluten can cause adverse reactions, so it is vital to be aware of how gluten-containing products might come into contact with gluten-free foods. This can occur in shared kitchen utensils, cooking surfaces, or even during the manufacturing process if gluten-free and gluten-containing foods are processed in the same facilities.

Being well-informed about these common sources of gluten helps in making safe food choices and maintaining a strict gluten-free diet. Regularly reviewing ingredient lists, opting for certified gluten-free products, and being mindful of cross-contamination are essential practices in ensuring that gluten is completely avoided. By understanding where gluten is commonly found, individuals can navigate their grocery shopping and meal preparation with greater confidence and precision.

Cross-Contamination and How to Avoid It

Cross-contamination is a crucial concern for anyone adhering to a gluten-free diet, as even minute traces of gluten can trigger adverse reactions. To prevent cross-contamination, it's essential to understand how it occurs and implement strategies to avoid it. Cross-contamination often happens when gluten-containing foods come into contact with gluten-free foods, either through shared utensils, cooking surfaces, or storage containers. This can occur at any stage, from food preparation to storage, making vigilance critical.

In the kitchen, start by ensuring that all cooking utensils, pots, and pans used for gluten-free foods are thoroughly cleaned and ideally dedicated solely to gluten-free cooking. This includes cutting boards, knives, and mixing bowls. Using separate utensils and surfaces for gluten-free foods minimizes the risk of gluten transfer. For example, if you prepare gluten-containing bread on a cutting board, be sure to clean the board thoroughly before using it for gluten-free foods.

Similarly, avoid using shared appliances such as toasters, which can harbor crumbs from gluten-containing bread. A dedicated toaster for gluten-free bread or other gluten-free items can be a worthwhile investment. When it comes to cooking, be cautious of items such as fryers and grills that may have been used for gluten-containing foods. The residue left behind can cross-contaminate gluten-free foods unless thoroughly cleaned or used exclusively for gluten-free purposes.

In terms of food storage, store gluten-free foods in separate, clearly labeled containers. This helps prevent accidental mixing of gluten-containing and gluten-free items. For instance, keep gluten-free pasta and cereals in their own containers and away from those containing gluten-containing products. Additionally, be mindful of bulk bins in stores, as gluten-free products scooped from these bins can be contaminated if the same scoops are used for gluten-containing items.

Cross-contamination can also occur outside the kitchen, particularly when eating out or ordering takeout. When dining at restaurants, communicate clearly with the staff about your gluten-free needs and inquire about their procedures for preventing cross-contamination. Opt for establishments that understand gluten-free requirements and have protocols in place to handle gluten-free foods separately from gluten-containing items.

When shopping, review the guide's section on reading labels carefully. Even products labeled as gluten-free can become contaminated if produced in facilities that handle gluten-containing ingredients. Check for certifications or statements indicating that the product was made in a dedicated gluten-free facility or that stringent cross-contamination measures are in place. This will help you choose products that align with your dietary needs.

Lastly, maintaining a gluten-free diet requires ongoing vigilance and education. As you become more familiar with cross-contamination risks and prevention strategies, you'll be better equipped to manage your gluten-free lifestyle. By consistently applying these practices and staying informed, you can protect yourself from accidental gluten exposure and enjoy the benefits of a well-managed gluten-free diet.

Chapter 2: Gluten-Free Foods to Eat

Fruits and Vegetables

Here's a detailed table covering fruits and vegetables that are naturally gluten-free, including instructions for their use, nutritional information, serving size, and cooking time:

Fruit/Vegetable	Instructions	Nutritional Information (per 1 cup serving)	Serving Size	Cooking Time
Apples	Wash and slice. Enjoy fresh or use in baking.	95 calories, 25g carbs, 4g fiber, 19g sugar, 0g protein	1 medium apple	N/A

Bananas	Peel and slice. Use fresh or in smoothies.	105 calories, 27g carbs, 3g fiber, 14g sugar, 1g protein	1 medium banana	N/A
Blueberries	Wash before use. Eat fresh or add to cereals.	84 calories, 21g carbs, 4g fiber, 15g sugar, 1g protein	1 cup	N/A
Carrots	Peel and cut into sticks or rounds. Use raw or cooked.	52 calories, 12g carbs, 3.5g fiber, 6g sugar, 1g protein	1 medium carrot	5-10 minutes (boiling)
Cucumbers	Wash and slice. Enjoy fresh in salads.	16 calories, 4g carbs, 1g fiber, 2g sugar, 1g protein	1 medium cucumber	N/A

Grapes	Wash and eat fresh. Can be frozen for a cool treat.	62 calories, 16g carbs, 1g fiber, 16g sugar, 0.5g protein	1 cup	N/A
Kale	Wash and chop. Use in salads or cook as a side.	33 calories, 6g carbs, 1.3g fiber, 0g sugar, 2g protein	1 cup chopped	5-10 minutes (steaming)
Oranges	Peel and segment. Eat fresh or use in juice.	62 calories, 15g carbs, 3g fiber, 12g sugar, 1g protein	1 medium orange	N/A
Peppers (Bell)	Wash, core, and slice. Use raw or	31 calories, 7g carbs, 2g fiber,	1 medium pepper	10-15 minutes (roasting)

	cook in dishes.	5g sugar, 1g protein		
Pineapple	Peel and core. Cut into chunks for fresh eating.	82 calories, 22g carbs, 2g fiber, 16g sugar, 1g protein	1 cup	N/A
Spinach	Wash thoroughl y. Use fresh in salads or cook.	7 calories, 1g carbs, 1g fiber, 0g sugar, 1g protein	1 cup cooked	2-5 minutes (steaming)
Strawberri es	Wash and hull. Eat fresh or add to desserts.	49 calories, 12g carbs, 3g fiber, 7g sugar, 1g protein	1 cup sliced	N/A
Sweet Potatoes	Peel and cut. Roast	103 calories, 24g carbs,	1 medium sweet potato	20-30 minutes (baking)

	or boil for dishes.	4g fiber, 7g sugar, 2g protein		
Tomatoes	Wash and slice. Use fresh in salads or cook.	22 calories, 5g carbs, 1.5g fiber, 3g sugar, 1g protein	1 medium tomato	N/A
Zucchini	Wash and slice. Use raw in salads or cook.	19 calories, 4g carbs, 1g fiber, 2g sugar, 1g protein	1 medium zucchini	5-10 minutes (sautéing)

This table provides a snapshot of how to prepare and enjoy various gluten-free fruits and vegetables, along with their nutritional benefits and cooking details.

Proteins

Here is a detailed table covering 15 gluten-free protein sources, including ingredients, instructions, nutritional information, serving size, and cooking time:

Protein Source	Ingredients	Instructions	Nutritional Information (per 3 oz serving)	Serving Size	Cooking Time
Chicken Breast	Skinless chicken breast	Season and grill or bake at 375°F for 25-30 minutes.	140 calories, 26g protein, 3g fat, 0g carbs	3 oz	25-30 minutes

| Salmon | Fresh salmon fillet | Season with salt, pepper, and lemon juice. Bake at 375°F for 15-20 minutes. | 200 calories, 22g protein, 13g fat, 0g carbs | 3 oz | 15-20 minutes |
| **Eggs** | Whole eggs | Boil, scramble, or fry. Boil for 10 minutes, scramble for 5 minutes, or fry for 3 | 210 calories, 18g protein, 15g fat, 1g carbs | 2 large eggs | 3-10 minutes |

		minutes.			
Tofu	Firm tofu	Marinate and pan-fry or bake at 375°F for 20-25 minutes.	70 calories, 8g protein, 4g fat, 2g carbs	3 oz	20-25 minutes
Ground Turkey	Ground turkey	Season and cook in a skillet over medium heat for 7-10 minutes, breaking up as	160 calories, 22g protein, 7g fat, 0g carbs	3 oz	7-10 minutes

		it cooks.			
Beef Sirloin	Sirloin steak	Season and grill or pan-sear for 4-5 minutes per side for medium-rare.	200 calories, 22g protein, 10g fat, 0g carbs	3 oz	8-10 minutes
Shrimp	Fresh or frozen shrimp	Peel and devein. Sauté in a skillet over medium-high heat for 3-4 minutes per side.	80 calories, 18g protein, 1g fat, 0g carbs	3 oz	6-8 minutes

Pork Tenderloin	Pork tenderloin	Season and roast at 375°F for 20-25 minutes or until internal temperature reaches 145°F.	150 calories, 22g protein, 6g fat, 0g carbs	3 oz	20-25 minutes
Cod	Fresh cod fillet	Season and bake at 375°F for 12-15 minutes or until fish flakes easily.	90 calories, 20g protein, 1g fat, 0g carbs	3 oz	12-15 minutes

Cottage Cheese	Low-fat cottage cheese	Eat as is or add to recipes.	80 calories, 11g protein, 1g fat, 6g carbs	1/2 cup	No cooking required
Chickpeas	Canned or cooked chickpeas	Rinse and drain. Use in salads, soups, or as a side dish.	130 calories, 6g protein, 2g fat, 22g carbs	1/2 cup	10 minutes
Lentils	Dry or canned lentils	Cook dry lentils in water for 20-25 minutes. Use canned	115 calories, 9g protein, 0g fat, 20g carbs	1/2 cup	20-25 minutes

		lentils directly.			
Edama me	Fresh or frozen edama me	Boil or steam for 5-7 minutes. Season with salt if desired.	120 calories, 11g protein, 5g fat, 9g carbs	1/2 cup	5-7 minutes
Quinoa	Quinoa grains	Rinse and cook in water for 15-20 minutes.	220 calories, 8g protein, 4g fat, 39g carbs	1/2 cup cooked	15-20 minutes
Greek Yogurt	Plain Greek yogurt	Eat as is or use in recipes.	100 calories, 10g protein, 0g fat, 6g carbs	1 cup	No cooking require d

This table provides a comprehensive overview of various gluten-free protein sources, offering practical guidance on preparation, nutritional details, and cooking times to help you maintain a balanced and enjoyable gluten-free diet.

Dairy and Dairy Alternatives

Here is a detailed table on dairy and dairy alternatives, including ingredients, instructions, nutritional information, serving size, and cooking time:

Ingredient	Instruction	Nutritional Information (per serving)	Serving Size	Cooking Time
Almond Milk	Shake well before use. Can be used in smoothies, cereals, or coffee.	Calories: 30, Protein: 1g, Carbs: 1g, Fat: 2.5g, Calcium: 450mg	1 cup	N/A
Coconut Milk	Shake before use. Suitable for cooking,	Calories: 45, Protein: 0g, Carbs: 1g, Fat: 4.5g,	1 cup	N/A

	baking, and as a beverage.	Calcium: 35mg		
Soy Milk	Shake well. Use in cooking, baking, and as a drink.	Calories: 80, Protein: 7g, Carbs: 4g, Fat: 4g, Calcium: 300mg	1 cup	N/A
Oat Milk	Shake well before use. Great in smoothies, coffee, and baking.	Calories: 60, Protein: 2g, Carbs: 11g, Fat: 1.5g, Calcium: 350mg	1 cup	N/A
Rice Milk	Shake before using. Ideal for drinking	Calories: 120, Protein: 1g, Carbs: 22g, Fat:	1 cup	N/A

	and cooking.	2.5g, Calcium: 300mg		
Cashew Milk	Shake well before use. Good in smoothies, coffee, or baking.	Calories: 25, Protein: 1g, Carbs: 1g, Fat: 2g, Calcium: 450mg	1 cup	N/A
Hemp Milk	Shake before using. Use in cereals, smoothies, or as a drink.	Calories: 60, Protein: 3g, Carbs: 0g, Fat: 5g, Calcium: 460mg	1 cup	N/A
Goat Milk	Use directly as a beverage or in cooking.	Calories: 168, Protein: 9g, Carbs: 11g, Fat:	1 cup	N/A

		10g, Calcium: 327mg		
Cow's Milk (Whole)	Use in cooking, baking, or as a drink.	Calories: 150, Protein: 8g, Carbs: 12g, Fat: 8g, Calcium: 291mg	1 cup	N/A
Cow's Milk (Skim)	Use in cooking, baking, or as a drink.	Calories: 90, Protein: 8g, Carbs: 12g, Fat: 0g, Calcium: 301mg	1 cup	N/A
Greek Yogurt (Plain)	Use as a snack or in recipes.	Calories: 100, Protein: 10g, Carbs: 6g,	1 cup	N/A

		Fat: 0g, Calcium: 110mg		
Almond Yogurt	Eat as a snack or breakfast option.	Calories: 60, Protein: 1g, Carbs: 6g, Fat: 3g, Calcium: 300mg	1 cup	N/A
Coconut Yogurt	Consume as a snack or breakfast.	Calories: 120, Protein: 1g, Carbs: 8g, Fat: 10g, Calcium: 0mg	1 cup	N/A
Soy Yogurt	Enjoy as a snack or in recipes.	Calories: 110, Protein: 6g, Carbs: 12g, Fat:	1 cup	N/A

		3g, Calcium: 300mg		
Kefir (Dairy)	Drink directly or use in smoothies.	Calories: 150, Protein: 9g, Carbs: 12g, Fat: 8g, Calcium: 300mg	1 cup	N/A

This table provides an overview of various dairy and dairy alternatives, including how to use them, their nutritional content, serving sizes, and whether any preparation or cooking time is required.

Grains and Starches

Here's a detailed table focusing on gluten-free grains and starches, including key information for each:

Ingredient	Instruction	Nutritional Information	Serving Size	Cooking Time
Rice	Rinse before cooking. Cook in a rice cooker or on the stove with water.	1 cup cooked: 205 calories, 0.4g fat, 44g carbs, 0.6g fiber, 4.3g protein	1 cup cooked	15-20 minutes
Quinoa	Rinse before cooking. Simmer in water or broth	1 cup cooked: 222 calories, 3.6g fat, 39g carbs,	1 cup cooked	15 minutes

			1 cup cooked	
	until tender.	5g fiber, 8g protein		
Millet	Rinse before cooking. Simmer in water until fluffy.	1 cup cooked: 207 calories, 1.7g fat, 41g carbs, 2.3g fiber, 6g protein	1 cup cooked	20 minutes
Buckwheat	Rinse before cooking. Simmer in water or broth until tender.	1 cup cooked: 155 calories, 1g fat, 33g carbs, 4.5g fiber, 6g protein	1 cup cooked	15 minutes
Amaranth	Rinse before cooking. Simmer in water	1 cup cooked: 251 calories, 4.2g fat, 46g carbs,	1 cup cooked	20 minutes

	until tender.	5g fiber, 9g protein		
Teff	Simmer in water until it forms a thick porridge.	1 cup cooked: 255 calories, 1.4g fat, 49g carbs, 7g fiber, 10g protein	1 cup cooked	15-20 minutes
Cornmea l	Cook in boiling water or milk, stirring until thickened.	1 cup cooked: 143 calories, 0.6g fat, 30g carbs, 2g fiber, 4g protein	1 cup cooked	10-15 minutes
Sorghum	Rinse before cooking. Simmer in water	1 cup cooked: 180 calories, 1g fat, 40g	1 cup cooked	30 minutes

	until tender.	carbs, 6g fiber, 6g protein		
Tapioca	Cook in water or milk until it becomes translucent and thick.	1 cup cooked: 200 calories, 0g fat, 50g carbs, 0g fiber, 0g protein	1 cup cooked	10-15 minutes
Arrowroot	Mix with water and cook until thickened.	1 cup cooked: 120 calories, 0g fat, 30g carbs, 0g fiber, 0g protein	1 cup cooked	5-10 minutes
Chia Seeds	Soak in water or milk until they form a gel-like	2 tablespoons: 120 calories, 7g fat, 12g	2 tablespoons	10 minutes (soaking)

	consistenc y.	carbs, 10g fiber, 4g protein		
Flaxseeds	Grind or soak before use.	2 tablespoo ns ground: 70 calories, 6g fat, 4g carbs, 4g fiber, 2g protein	2 tablespoo ns	5 minutes (soaking)
Oats (Certifie d Gluten-F ree)	Cook in water or milk until tender.	1 cup cooked: 154 calories, 3g fat, 27g carbs, 4g fiber, 6g protein	1 cup cooked	5-10 minutes
Hemp Seeds	Sprinkle on salads, yogurt, or	2 tablespoo ns: 110	2 tablespoo ns	No cooking needed

	blend into smoothies .	calories, 9g fat, 1g carbs, 1g fiber, 6g protein		

This table provides a comprehensive look at various gluten-free grains and starches, highlighting their preparation methods, nutritional content, typical serving sizes, and cooking times to help you make informed choices for your gluten-free diet.

Nuts and Seeds

Here is a detailed comprehensive table about nuts and seeds, including information on ingredients, instructions, nutritional information, serving size, and cooking time.

Ingredient	Instructions	Nutritional Information (per 1 oz)	Serving Size	Cooking Time
Almonds	Eat raw or roasted. For roasting, bake at 350°F for 10-12 minutes.	Calories: 160, Protein: 6g, Fat: 14g, Carbs: 6g, Fiber: 3g	1 oz (28g)	10-12 minutes (roasting)
Walnuts	Eat raw or toasted. Toast at 350°F for 8-10 minutes.	Calories: 185, Protein: 4g, Fat: 18g,	1 oz (28g)	8-10 minutes (toasting)

		Carbs: 4g, Fiber: 2g		
Cashews	Eat raw or roasted. Roast at 350°F for 10-15 minutes.	Calories: 155, Protein: 5g, Fat: 12g, Carbs: 9g, Fiber: 1g	1 oz (28g)	10-15 minutes (roasting)
Pecans	Eat raw or roasted. Roast at 350°F for 8-10 minutes.	Calories: 200, Protein: 3g, Fat: 21g, Carbs: 4g, Fiber: 3g	1 oz (28g)	8-10 minutes (roasting)
Pistachios	Eat raw or roasted. Roast at 350°F for 8-10 minutes.	Calories: 160, Protein: 6g, Fat: 13g, Carbs: 8g, Fiber: 3g	1 oz (28g)	8-10 minutes (roasting)

Sunflower Seeds	Eat raw or roasted. Roast at 350°F for 10-15 minutes.	Calories: 165, Protein: 6g, Fat: 14g, Carbs: 6g, Fiber: 2g	1 oz (28g)	10-15 minutes (roasting)
Chia Seeds	Eat raw, soaked in liquid, or blended. Can also be toasted for added crunch.	Calories: 138, Protein: 5g, Fat: 9g, Carbs: 12g, Fiber: 10g	1 oz (28g)	0 minutes (raw); 2-3 minutes (toasting)
Flaxseeds	Eat raw, ground, or toasted. For toasting, heat in a dry skillet over medium	Calories: 150, Protein: 5g, Fat: 12g, Carbs: 8g, Fiber: 8g	1 oz (28g)	5 minutes (toasting)

	heat for 5 minutes.			
Pumpkin Seeds	Eat raw or roasted. Roast at 350°F for 10-15 minutes.	Calories: 151, Protein: 7g, Fat: 13g, Carbs: 5g, Fiber: 1g	1 oz (28g)	10-15 minutes (roasting)
Hemp Seeds	Eat raw or sprinkled on dishes. Can also be blended into smoothies.	Calories: 160, Protein: 10g, Fat: 14g, Carbs: 2g, Fiber: 1g	1 oz (28g)	0 minutes (raw)
Brazil Nuts	Eat raw or roasted. Roast at 350°F for 8-10 minutes.	Calories: 190, Protein: 4g, Fat: 19g,	1 oz (28g)	8-10 minutes (roasting)

		Carbs: 4g, Fiber: 2g		
Macadamia Nuts	Eat raw or roasted. Roast at 350°F for 10-12 minutes.	Calories: 204, Protein: 2g, Fat: 21g, Carbs: 4g, Fiber: 2g	1 oz (28g)	10-12 minutes (roasting)
Hazelnuts	Eat raw or toasted. Toast at 350°F for 10-12 minutes.	Calories: 178, Protein: 4g, Fat: 17g, Carbs: 5g, Fiber: 3g	1 oz (28g)	10-12 minutes (toasting)
Pine Nuts	Eat raw or toasted. Toast at 350°F for 5-7 minutes.	Calories: 191, Protein: 4g, Fat: 20g, Carbs: 4g, Fiber: 1g	1 oz (28g)	5-7 minutes (toasting)

| Sesame Seeds | Eat raw or toasted. Toast at 350°F for 6-8 minutes. | Calories: 160, Protein: 5g, Fat: 14g, Carbs: 6g, Fiber: 3g | 1 oz (28g) | 6-8 minutes (toasting) |

This table provides a comprehensive overview of popular nuts and seeds, including their preparation methods, nutritional profiles, typical serving sizes, and cooking times.

Oils and Fats

Here is a detailed table on oils and fats, including key information for each item:

Ingredient	Description	Nutritional Information (per 1 tablespoon)	Serving Size	Cooking Time
Olive Oil	A versatile oil with a rich, fruity flavor, great for sautéing and dressings.	119 calories, 14g fat (2g saturated), 0g carbs, 0g protein	1 tablespoon	Varies by recipe
Coconut Oil	Solid at room temperature, ideal	117 calories, 14g fat (12g	1 tablespoon	3-5 minutes for

	for baking and high-heat cooking.	saturated), 0g carbs, 0g protein		medium heat
Avocado Oil	High smoke point oil, excellent for frying and grilling.	124 calories, 14g fat (2g saturated), 0g carbs, 0g protein	1 tablespoon	Varies by recipe
Canola Oil	Mild flavor, good for frying and baking.	124 calories, 14g fat (1g saturated), 0g carbs, 0g protein	1 tablespoon	Varies by recipe
Grapesee d Oil	Light oil with a high smoke point, suitable	120 calories, 14g fat (1g saturated)	1 tablespoon	Varies by recipe

	for sautéing and dressings.	, 0g carbs, 0g protein		
Sunflowe r Oil	Mild flavor, commonl y used for frying and baking.	120 calories, 14g fat (1g saturated) , 0g carbs, 0g protein	1 tablespoo n	Varies by recipe
Safflower Oil	High smoke point, ideal for frying and stir-frying.	120 calories, 14g fat (1g saturated) , 0g carbs, 0g protein	1 tablespoo n	Varies by recipe
Sesame Oil	Strong flavor, used for stir-frying and dressings.	120 calories, 14g fat (2g saturated)	1 tablespoo n	Varies by recipe

		, 0g carbs, 0g protein		
Walnut Oil	Nutty flavor, best for drizzling and salad dressings.	120 calories, 13g fat (1g saturated), 0g carbs, 0g protein	1 tablespoon	Varies by recipe
Flaxseed Oil	High in omega-3s, used mainly in dressings and smoothies.	120 calories, 14g fat (1g saturated), 0g carbs, 0g protein	1 tablespoon	Not used for cooking
Hemp Oil	Nutty flavor, rich in essential fatty acids, used in	120 calories, 14g fat (1g saturated), 0g carbs, 0g protein	1 tablespoon	Not used for cooking

	dressings and dips.			
Pumpkin Seed Oil	Earthy flavor, ideal for finishing dishes and dressings.	120 calories, 14g fat (2g saturated), 0g carbs, 0g protein	1 tablespoon	Not used for cooking
MCT Oil	Medium-chain triglycerides, used in smoothies and dressings.	115 calories, 14g fat (0g saturated), 0g carbs, 0g protein	1 tablespoon	Not used for cooking
Butter	Classic cooking fat, used for baking and sautéing.	102 calories, 12g fat (7g saturated), 0g carbs, 0g protein	1 tablespoon	Varies by recipe

| **Ghee** | Clarified butter with a higher smoke point, ideal for high-heat cooking. | 134 calories, 15g fat (9g saturated), 0g carbs, 0g protein | 1 tablespoon | Varies by recipe |

This table provides a comprehensive overview of various oils and fats, including their descriptions, nutritional information, typical serving sizes, and cooking times where applicable. This information helps in selecting suitable options for different gluten-free cooking needs.

Beverages

Here is a detailed table for "Beverages" in relation to a gluten-free diet:

Beverage	Ingredients	Instructions	Nutritional Information	Serving Size	Cooking Time
Green Tea	Green tea leaves, water	Steep 1 teaspoon of green tea leaves in 8 ounces of boiling water for 2-3 minutes. Strain and serve.	0 calories, 0g fat, 0g carbs, 0g protein	8 ounces	3 minutes

| Black Coffee | Ground coffee, water | Brew 1-2 tablespoons of coffee grounds in 8 ounces of water using a coffee maker or French press. | 2 calories, 0g fat, 0g carbs, 0g protein | 8 ounces | 5 minutes |
| Herbal Tea | Herbal tea bag, water | Steep 1 herbal tea bag in 8 ounces of boiling water for 5 minutes | Varies by herb; typically 0 calories | 8 ounces | 5 minutes |

		. Remove the bag and serve.			
Almond Milk	Almonds, water, sweetener (optional)	Blend 1 cup of soaked almonds with 2-3 cups of water. Strain through a cheesecloth. Sweeten if desired.	30 calories, 2.5g fat, 1g carbs, 1g protein	1 cup	10 minutes
Soy Milk	Soybeans, water, sweeten	Soak 1 cup of soybeans	80 calories, 4g fat, 4g	1 cup	20 minutes

| | er (optional) | overnight. Blend with 4 cups of water. Strain through cheesecloth. Sweeten if desired. | carbs, 7g protein | | |
| **Coconut Water** | Coconut water | Chill and serve. Can be consumed directly from the container. | 45 calories, 0g fat, 11g carbs, 1g protein | 8 ounces | 0 minutes |

| Fruit Juice | Fresh fruit, water, sweetener (optional) | Juice fresh fruits or use pre-packaged, ensuring no gluten-containing additives. | Varies by fruit; typically 100 calories | 8 ounces | 5 minutes |
| Lemonade | Lemon juice, water, sugar | Mix 1 cup of lemon juice with 4 cups of water. Add 1 cup of sugar. Stir until | 100 calories, 0g fat, 26g carbs, 0g protein | 8 ounces | 5 minutes |

		dissolved.			
Smoothie	Fresh fruit, yogurt, ice	Blend 1 cup of fresh fruit with 1/2 cup of yogurt and 1/2 cup of ice until smooth.	150 calories, 2g fat, 25g carbs, 5g protein	8 ounces	5 minutes
Sparkling Water	Carbonated water	Chill and serve plain or with a slice of lemon or lime.	0 calories, 0g fat, 0g carbs, 0g protein	8 ounces	0 minutes

Chai Tea	Black tea, spices (cinnamon, cardamom, etc.), milk	Brew black tea with spices. Add milk and sweetener if desired.	60 calories, 2g fat, 10g carbs, 2g protein	8 ounces	10 minutes
Hot Chocolate	Cocoa powder, milk, sugar	Mix 2 tablespoons of cocoa powder with 1 cup of milk and 2 tablespoons of sugar. Heat until warm.	190 calories, 8g fat, 24g carbs, 6g protein	8 ounces	5 minutes

| Kombucha | Tea, sugar, SCOBY (symbiotic culture of bacteria and yeast) | Brew tea, add sugar, and ferment with SCOBY for 7-14 days. | 30 calories, 0g fat, 8g carbs, 0g protein | 8 ounces | 7 days |
| Rice Milk | Rice, water, sweetener (optional) | Blend 1 cup of cooked rice with 4 cups of water. Strain through a cheesecloth. Sweeten if desired. | 120 calories, 2.5g fat, 23g carbs, 1g protein | 1 cup | 10 minutes |

| **Oat Milk** | Oats, water, sweetener (optional) | Blend 1 cup of oats with 4 cups of water. Strain through a cheesecloth. Sweeten if desired. | 60 calories, 1.5g fat, 10g carbs, 2g protein | 1 cup | 10 minutes |

This table provides a comprehensive overview of gluten-free beverages, including their ingredients, instructions, nutritional information, serving sizes, and preparation times.

Snacks

Here's a detailed table for gluten-free snacks, including ingredients, instructions, nutritional information, serving size, and cooking time:

Snack	Ingredients	Instructions	Nutritional Information (per serving)	Serving Size	Cooking Time
1. Almond Joy Energy Balls	1 cup almonds, 1 cup pitted dates, 1/2 cup unsweetened shredded coconut, 2 tbsp	Blend all ingredients in a food processor until combined. Roll into balls.	Calories: 180, Fat: 12g, Carbs: 20g, Protein: 4g	2 balls	10 minutes

	cocoa powder				
2. Apple Slices with Peanut Butter	1 apple, 2 tbsp peanut butter, 1 tbsp honey (optional)	Slice the apple and spread peanut butter on each slice. Drizzle with honey if desired.	Calories: 160, Fat: 8g, Carbs: 22g, Protein: 4g	1 apple	5 minutes
3. Rice Cakes with Avocado	2 rice cakes, 1 ripe avocado, 1 tbsp lemon juice, salt and pepper	Mash avocado with lemon juice, salt, and pepper. Spread	Calories: 150, Fat: 10g, Carbs: 15g, Protein: 2g	2 rice cakes	5 minutes

		on rice cakes.			
4. Greek Yogurt with Berries	1 cup Greek yogurt, 1/2 cup mixed berries, 1 tbsp honey	Combine Greek yogurt with berries and honey. Stir until mixed.	Calories: 180, Fat: 4g, Carbs: 25g, Protein: 12g	1 cup	5 minutes
5. Carrot and Celery Sticks with Hummus	1 cup carrot sticks, 1 cup celery sticks, 1/2 cup hummus	Serve carrot and celery sticks with hummus for dipping.	Calories: 100, Fat: 5g, Carbs: 12g, Protein: 3g	1 cup of each	5 minutes

| 6. **Home made Trail Mix** | 1/2 cup almonds, 1/2 cup walnuts, 1/4 cup dried cranberries, 1/4 cup pumpkin seeds | Mix all ingredients in a bowl. Store in an airtight container. | Calories: 200, Fat: 15g, Carbs: 15g, Protein: 6g | 1/4 cup | 5 minutes |
| 7. **Baked Sweet Potato Chips** | 2 medium sweet potatoes, 2 tbsp olive oil, salt and pepper | Slice sweet potatoes thinly, toss with olive oil, salt, and pepper. Bake at 400°F | Calories: 150, Fat: 7g, Carbs: 25g, Protein: 2g | 1 cup | 25 minutes |

		for 20 minutes, flipping halfway.			
8. Chia Seed Pudding	1/4 cup chia seeds, 1 cup almond milk, 1 tbsp maple syrup, 1/2 tsp vanilla extract	Mix chia seeds with almond milk, maple syrup, and vanilla extract. Refrigerate for at least 2 hours or overnight.	Calories: 150, Fat: 8g, Carbs: 15g, Protein: 4g	1/2 cup	10 minutes prep, 2+ hours refrigeration
9. Edama	1 cup shelled	Steam edama	Calories: 120,	1 cup	10 minutes

me with Sea Salt	edamame, 1 tsp sea salt	me until tender. Sprinkle with sea salt.	Fat: 5g, Carbs: 10g, Protein: 11g		
10. Quinoa Salad	1 cup cooked quinoa, 1/2 cup cherry tomatoes, 1/4 cup diced cucumber, 2 tbsp olive oil, 1 tbsp lemon juice	Mix all ingredients in a bowl. Stir until combined.	Calories: 200, Fat: 10g, Carbs: 25g, Protein: 6g	1 cup	10 minutes
11. Cottag	1 cup cottage	Combine	Calories: 150,	1 cup	5 minutes

e Cheese with Pineapple	cheese, 1/2 cup pineapple chunks	cottage cheese and pineapple chunks in a bowl. Stir until mixed.	Fat: 2g, Carbs: 18g, Protein: 12g		
12. Gluten-Free Crackers with Cheese	6 gluten-free crackers, 2 oz cheese (e.g., cheddar or gouda)	Arrange cheese slices on crackers.	Calories: 200, Fat: 15g, Carbs: 10g, Protein: 10g	6 crackers	5 minutes
13. Smoothie with	1 banana, 1 cup spinach	Blend all ingredients	Calories: 180, Fat: 2g, Carbs:	1 cup	5 minutes

Spinach and Banana	, 1 cup almond milk, 1 tbsp honey	until smooth.	36g, Protein: 4g		
14. Popcorn with Nutritional Yeast	1 cup popcorn, 2 tbsp nutritional yeast, 1 tbsp olive oil	Pop popcorn. Toss with nutritional yeast and olive oil.	Calories: 120, Fat: 4g, Carbs: 20g, Protein: 4g	1 cup	10 minutes
15. Roasted Chickpeas	1 can chickpeas, 2 tbsp olive oil, 1 tsp paprika, salt to taste	Rinse and drain chickpeas. Toss with olive oil, paprika, and	Calories: 150, Fat: 6g, Carbs: 20g, Protein: 6g	1/2 cup	30 minutes

		salt. Roast at 400°F for 25 minutes , stirring halfway.			

This table provides a variety of gluten-free snack options, along with their preparation details, nutritional content, and cooking times, helping you stay informed and make healthy choices for your gluten-free diet.

Chapter 3: Foods to Avoid

Grains and Cereals

Here's a detailed table about "Grains and Cereals" (Foods to Avoid) in relation to a gluten-free grocery list and food, including why each grain and cereal should be avoided:

Grain/Cereal	Description	Reason to Avoid
Wheat	A staple grain used in many breads, pastas, and baked goods.	Contains gluten, which can cause severe digestive issues and other health problems for people with celiac disease or gluten intolerance.
Barley	Commonly used in soups, stews, and beer.	Contains gluten, and even small amounts can trigger symptoms in those with

		gluten sensitivity or celiac disease.
Rye	Often found in bread and crackers, especially rye bread.	Contains gluten, and its consumption can lead to adverse health effects for individuals with gluten-related disorders.
Triticale	A hybrid of wheat and rye, used in similar applications to wheat and rye.	Contains gluten, making it unsuitable for gluten-free diets.
Spelt	An ancient grain related to wheat, used in various baked goods and pastas.	Contains gluten and can cause the same reactions as other gluten-containing grains for those with gluten intolerance or celiac disease.

Kamut	Another ancient grain similar to wheat, used in breads and cereals.	Contains gluten, making it inappropriate for a gluten-free diet.
Farro	A type of wheat often used in salads and soups.	Contains gluten and should be avoided by those who need to adhere to a gluten-free diet.
Bulgur	Cracked wheat commonly used in Middle Eastern dishes like tabbouleh.	Contains gluten, posing a risk to individuals with gluten sensitivity or celiac disease.
Semolina	A coarse flour made from durum wheat, used in pasta and couscous.	Contains gluten, which can cause health issues for those with celiac disease or gluten intolerance.
Durum Wheat	A hard variety of wheat used to	Contains gluten, making it

	make pasta and bread.	unsuitable for those on a gluten-free diet.
Einkorn	An ancient wheat variety used in baking and cooking.	Contains gluten, and its consumption can lead to adverse reactions in those with gluten-related disorders.
Freekeh	Young, green wheat that is roasted and used in salads and side dishes.	Contains gluten, making it inappropriate for gluten-free diets.
Emmer	Another ancient wheat variety used in breads and pastas.	Contains gluten, which can cause issues for individuals with celiac disease or gluten sensitivity.
Couscous	Small granules made from durum	Contains gluten, posing a risk to

| | wheat, used as a side dish or in salads. | those with gluten-related health problems. |
| **Barley Malt** | Used as a flavoring and sweetener in various products, including cereals and beverages. | Contains gluten and should be avoided by those who need to follow a gluten-free diet. |

This table helps identify grains and cereals that must be avoided on a gluten-free diet, explaining the reasons why each one is unsuitable. This information is crucial for those managing gluten intolerance or celiac disease, ensuring they can make safe and informed dietary choices.

Processed Foods

Here's a detailed table for processed foods to avoid on a gluten-free diet, including reasons why each should be avoided:

Processed Food	Reason to Avoid
Packaged Snacks (e.g., crackers, cookies)	Many packaged snacks contain wheat flour, barley malt, or other gluten-containing ingredients as thickeners or flavorings.
Breaded and Battered Foods	Breaded or battered items, such as chicken nuggets or fish sticks, are typically coated with wheat flour or breadcrumbs.
Processed Meats (e.g., sausages, deli meats)	These can contain fillers, binders, or flavorings made from gluten-containing grains.
Canned Soups and Broths	Many canned soups and broths use wheat flour or

	barley malt as a thickener or flavor enhancer.
Salad Dressings and Sauces	Certain dressings and sauces, including soy sauce, contain gluten as a thickener or flavoring agent.
Seasoned Snack Foods (e.g., chips)	Seasoned snacks often contain gluten in the seasoning or as a binder to help flavors adhere to the snack.
Breakfast Cereals	Many cereals contain wheat, barley malt, or oats that are contaminated with gluten during processing.
Beer and Malt Beverages	These beverages are brewed with barley or wheat, which contain gluten.
Pre-Made Meals and Frozen Dinners	These meals often include sauces, gravies, or breaded items containing gluten.

Certain Candies and Sweets	Some candies use wheat flour or barley malt for texture or flavor.
Gravies and Sauces	Many gravies and sauces use wheat flour as a thickener.
Instant Noodles and Pasta	Instant noodles and pasta are typically made from wheat flour.
Energy and Granola Bars	These bars often contain oats that are not certified gluten-free, or they use wheat as a binder.
Processed Cheese Products	Some processed cheeses use gluten-containing ingredients for flavor or texture.
Imitation Seafood (e.g., imitation crab)	Imitation seafood often contains fillers or binders derived from wheat or other gluten-containing grains.

This table outlines various processed foods that should be avoided on a gluten-free diet, along with the reasons for their avoidance. By understanding which foods contain hidden sources of gluten, you can make informed choices and maintain a strict gluten-free lifestyle.

Hidden Sources of Gluten

Here's a detailed table for "Hidden Sources of Gluten" including why you should avoid each source:

Hidden Source of Gluten	Description	Why You Should Avoid It
Malt and Malt Extract	Derived from barley, malt and malt extract are commonly used in cereals, candies, and beverages.	Barley contains gluten, and these derivatives can cause reactions in those with gluten sensitivity or celiac disease.
Modified Food Starch	Often made from wheat, modified food starch is used as a thickener in soups, sauces, and processed foods.	Unless specified as corn or another gluten-free source, it can introduce gluten into your diet, leading to health issues.
Soy Sauce	Traditional soy sauce is brewed using wheat.	Even small amounts can lead to gluten exposure,

		causing symptoms in sensitive individuals.
Bouillon Cubes and Broths	Many commercial bouillons and broths contain gluten-based additives or thickeners.	These hidden sources can compromise a gluten-free diet, leading to unintended gluten consumption.
Imitation Seafood	Often made with wheat-containing fillers and flavorings.	These fillers can introduce gluten into what might otherwise be a gluten-free dish, posing a risk for those with gluten intolerance.
Processed Meats	Sausages, hot dogs, and deli meats may contain gluten as fillers or binders.	Gluten additives are common in processed meats, making it essential to check labels to

		avoid inadvertent gluten intake.
Salad Dressings and Marinades	Some dressings and marinades use gluten-containing thickeners or flavorings.	These hidden sources can easily be overlooked, leading to unintentional gluten exposure and health complications.
Seasoned Rice and Pasta Mixes	Often contain gluten-based seasonings or flavor packets.	Gluten additives in the seasoning can contaminate an otherwise gluten-free food, making it unsafe for those with gluten sensitivities.
Gravy Mixes and Sauces	Frequently thickened with wheat flour or other gluten-containing ingredients.	These mixes can introduce gluten into meals, posing a risk for gluten-sensitive individuals.

Veggie Burgers and Meat Substitutes	Some meat substitutes use wheat gluten as a protein source or binding agent.	These products can be deceptive, as they might seem gluten-free but contain significant amounts of gluten.
Candy and Sweets	Some candies use gluten-containing ingredients for texture or flavoring.	Gluten additives in candies can lead to accidental gluten consumption, which is particularly concerning for children with gluten sensitivities.
Pre-Packaged Spices and Seasonings	Gluten is sometimes used as an anti-caking agent or filler.	These hidden sources can contaminate your meals, making it essential to choose certified gluten-free spices and seasonings.

Beer and Certain Alcohols	Beer is brewed with barley, and some flavored alcoholic beverages contain gluten.	Even small amounts of gluten in these drinks can trigger symptoms, making it necessary to choose gluten-free labeled alcoholic beverages.
French Fries (in some restaurants)	French fries may be fried in the same oil as gluten-containing foods or coated in gluten-based batter.	Cross-contamination in fryers can introduce gluten into your meal, which can be harmful to those with celiac disease or gluten intolerance.
Instant Coffee and Drinks	Some instant coffee and drink mixes use gluten-containing fillers or flavorings.	These hidden sources can lead to unintended gluten exposure, affecting your overall health and well-being.

This table highlights various hidden sources of gluten and explains why avoiding them is crucial for maintaining a gluten-free diet. Understanding these hidden sources can help you make informed choices and prevent accidental gluten consumption.

Cross-Contaminated Foods

Here is a detailed table about "Cross-Contaminated Foods" (Foods to Avoid) in relation to a gluten-free grocery list and food:

Cross-Contaminated Food	Why You Should Avoid It
Oats (unless certified gluten-free)	Oats are often grown, harvested, and processed alongside wheat, barley, and rye, leading to cross-contamination. Always choose oats labeled as gluten-free to ensure they are safe.
French Fries (from shared fryers)	Fries cooked in the same oil as breaded items can become contaminated with gluten. Opt for fries cooked in dedicated gluten-free fryers.
Deli Meats (sliced on shared equipment)	Slicers and counters used for both gluten-containing and gluten-free products can transfer gluten. Look for

	pre-packaged, gluten-free labeled deli meats.
Condiments (e.g., butter, jam, mayonnaise)	Shared jars can introduce crumbs from gluten-containing bread. Use separate containers for gluten-free items or single-serving packets.
Bulk Bins (grains, nuts, seeds)	Scoops and bins may be shared between gluten and non-gluten products, leading to contamination. Purchase pre-packaged gluten-free products instead.
Communal Snacks (e.g., chips, pretzels)	Bowls of snacks shared at parties can be contaminated by people reaching in with hands that have touched gluten-containing foods. Opt for individually packaged snacks.
Ice Cream (scooped in shared containers)	Ice cream parlors may use the same scoop for multiple

	flavors, risking cross-contamination. Choose pre-packaged ice cream labeled gluten-free.
Sushi (with shared preparation surfaces)	Sushi prepared on the same surfaces as other foods containing gluten (e.g., tempura) can be contaminated. Request sushi made with clean equipment or choose restaurants with gluten-free protocols.
Salad Bars (shared utensils)	Utensils and surfaces in salad bars can cross-contaminate gluten-free items with gluten-containing ingredients. Opt for pre-packaged salads labeled gluten-free.
Marinated Meats (with shared marinades)	Marinades used for both gluten-containing and gluten-free meats can cross-contaminate. Choose plain, unmarinated meats or

	verify the marinade is gluten-free.
Breakfast Buffets (e.g., toasters, waffle makers)	Shared equipment at buffets can introduce gluten to gluten-free items. Avoid using communal toasters or waffle makers unless they are dedicated gluten-free.
Soup (from shared pots)	Soup served from shared pots can become contaminated if one contains gluten. Ensure the soup is prepared in a dedicated gluten-free pot or opt for packaged gluten-free soup.
Pizza (prepared in shared ovens)	Pizza baked in the same oven as gluten-containing pizzas can be contaminated. Choose pizza from establishments with dedicated gluten-free ovens or preparation areas.
Cereals (from shared dispensers)	Dispensers that handle both gluten-containing and

	gluten-free cereals can lead to cross-contamination. Select pre-packaged gluten-free cereals.
Seasonings and Spices (from shared containers)	Shared spice containers can introduce gluten if spoons or hands contaminated with gluten touch them. Use dedicated gluten-free spices or single-use packets.

Understanding and avoiding these cross-contaminated foods is vital for maintaining a strict gluten-free diet.

Cross-contamination can occur at various stages of food handling, from harvesting and processing to preparation and serving. By being aware of these risks and choosing foods that are clearly labeled and prepared in gluten-free environments, you can minimize the risk of accidental gluten exposure and ensure your diet remains safe and healthy.

Conclusion

Embracing a gluten-free lifestyle can initially seem daunting, but with the right tools and information, it becomes a manageable and rewarding journey. The "Gluten-Free Grocery List and Food" guide serves as an invaluable resource, providing clarity and confidence in navigating a gluten-free diet. By understanding which foods are safe and which to avoid, you can make informed choices that support your health and well-being.

The guide emphasizes the importance of meticulous label reading and awareness of potential cross-contamination. These skills are essential for avoiding hidden sources of gluten that can easily find their way into your meals. With practice, these habits become second nature, allowing you to enjoy a diverse and satisfying diet without fear of accidental gluten exposure.

A well-rounded gluten-free diet includes a variety of fruits, vegetables, proteins, grains, and dairy alternatives, all of which are detailed in the guide. By incorporating these foods into your daily meals, you ensure that your diet remains balanced and nutritious. The guide also provides practical tips on meal planning and budgeting, helping you maintain a gluten-free diet that is both affordable and enjoyable.

Cross-contamination is a significant concern for anyone on a gluten-free diet, but the guide offers comprehensive strategies to mitigate this risk. From dedicated cooking utensils and appliances to careful food storage practices, these measures help create a safe kitchen environment. Additionally, the guide's advice on dining out and choosing gluten-free products further safeguards against unintentional gluten consumption.

The detailed lists of gluten-free snacks, meals, and recommended brands make grocery shopping a less overwhelming experience. With these resources at your disposal, you can quickly identify safe products and explore new food options. This not only simplifies shopping but also expands your culinary horizons, making a gluten-free diet more enjoyable and less restrictive.

Using the "Gluten-Free Grocery List and Food" guide as a continuous reference ensures that you stay updated on the best practices and newest products in the gluten-free market. As the food industry evolves, new gluten-free options become available, and staying informed helps you make the best choices for your health. The guide's ongoing relevance and practicality make it a vital tool in your gluten-free journey.

Incorporating these practices into your daily routine will lead to a more confident and fulfilling gluten-free lifestyle. The guide empowers you with the knowledge and resources needed to navigate dietary challenges and embrace a healthier way of living. With each step, you build a stronger foundation for long-term wellness and enjoyment of gluten-free foods.